Mediterranean S Budge

Super-Quick and Healthy Snacks Recipes to Boost Your Lifestyle and Save Money

Fern Bullock

Table of Contents

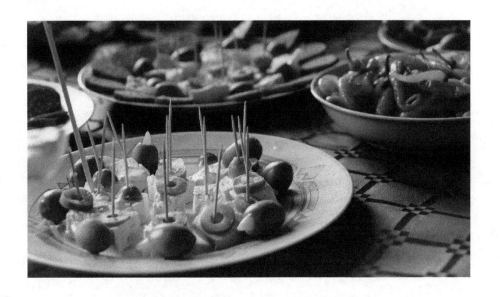

Kale Spread

Prep time: 10 minutes I **Cooking time:** 20 minutes I

Servings: 4

Ingredients:

- 1 bunch kale leaves
- 1 cup coconut cream
- 1 shallot, chopped
- 1 tablespoon olive oil
- 1 teaspoon chili powder
- A pinch of black pepper

Directions:

1. Heat up a pan with the oil over medium heat, add the shallots, stir and sauté for 4 minutes.
2. Add the kale and the other ingredients, bring to a simmer and cook over medium heat for 16 minutes.
3. Blend using an immersion blender, divide into bowls and serve as a snack.

Nutrition facts per serving: calories 188, fat 17.9, fiber 2.1, carbs 7.6, protein 2.5

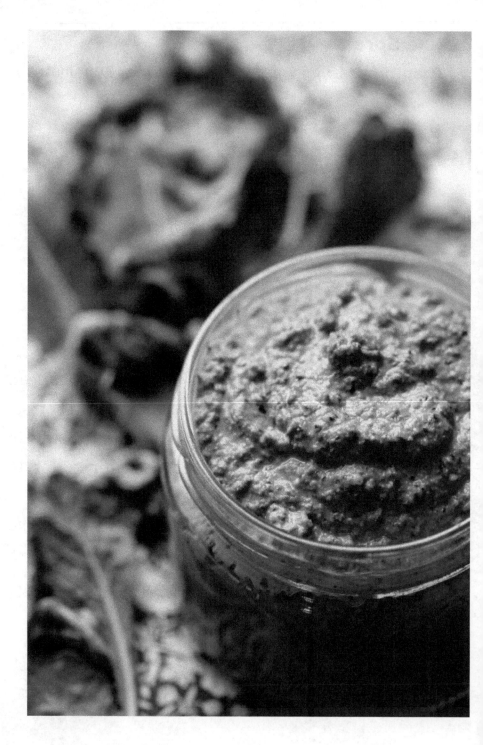

Garlic Beets Bites

Prep time: 10 minutes I **Cooking time:** 35 minutes I

Servings: 4

Ingredients:

- 2 beets, peeled and thinly sliced
- 1 tablespoon avocado oil
- 1 teaspoon cumin, ground
- 1 teaspoon fennel seeds, crushed
- 2 teaspoons garlic, minced

Directions:

1. Spread the beet chips on a lined baking sheet, add the oil and the other ingredients, toss, introduce in the oven and bake at 400 degrees F for 35 minutes.
2. Divide into bowls and serve as a snack.

Nutrition facts per serving: calories 32, fat 0.7, fiber 1.4, carbs 6.1, protein 1.1

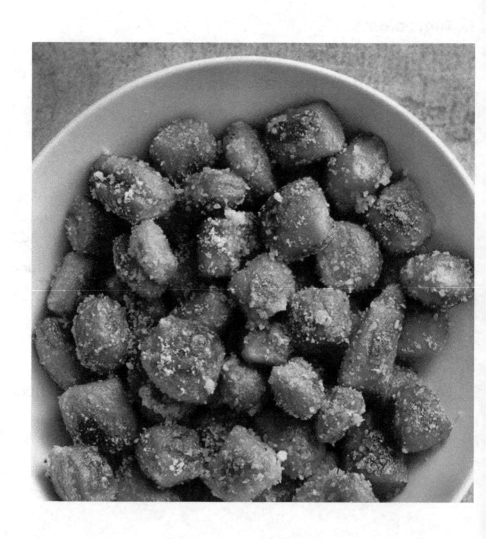

Yogurt Zucchini Dip

Prep time: 5 minutes I **Cooking time:** 10 minutes I

Servings: 4

Ingredients:

- ½ cup nonfat yogurt
- 2 zucchinis, chopped
- 1 tablespoon olive oil
- 2 spring onions, chopped
- ¼ cup veggie stock
- 2 garlic cloves, minced
- 1 tablespoon dill, chopped
- A pinch of nutmeg, ground

Directions:

1. Heat up a pan with the oil over medium heat, add the onions and garlic, stir and sauté for 3 minutes.
2. Add the zucchinis and the other ingredients except the yogurt, toss, cook for 7 minutes more and take off the heat.
3. Add the yogurt, blend using an immersion blender, divide into bowls and serve.

Nutrition facts per serving: calories 76, fat 4.1, fiber 1.5, carbs 7.2, protein 3.4

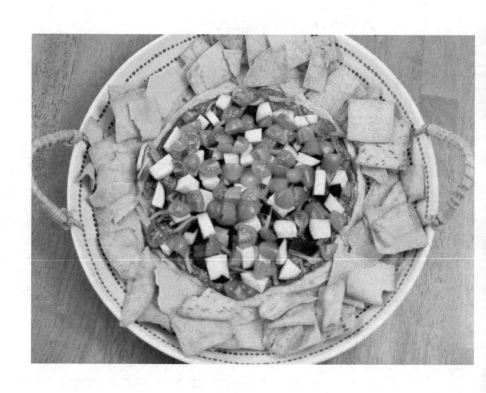

Apple Bites

Prep time: 10 minutes I **Cooking time:** 20 minutes I
Servings: 4

Ingredients:

- 2 tablespoons olive oil
- 1 teaspoon smoked paprika
- 1 cup sunflower seeds
- 1 cup chia seeds
- 2 apples, cored and cut into wedges
- ½ teaspoon cumin, ground
- A pinch of cayenne pepper

Directions:

1. In a bowl, combine the seeds with the apples and the other ingredients, toss, spread on a lined baking sheet, introduce in the oven and bake at 350 degrees F for 20 minutes.
2. Divide into bowls and serve as a snack.

Nutrition facts per serving: calories 222, fat 15.4, fiber 6.4, carbs 21.1, protein 4

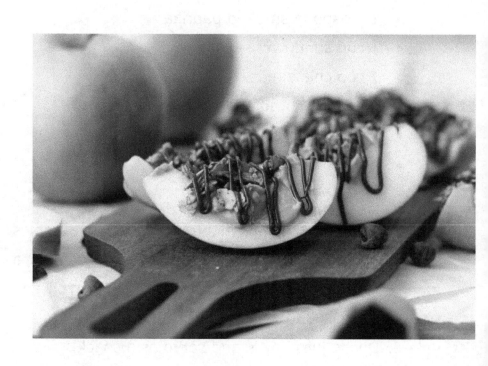

Pumpkin and Lemon Dip

Prep time: 5 minutes I **Cooking time:** 0 minutes I

Servings: 4

Ingredients:

- 2 cups pumpkin flesh
- ½ cup pumpkin seeds
- 1 tablespoon lemon juice
- 1 tablespoon sesame seed paste
- 1 tablespoon olive oil

Directions:

1. In a blender, combine the pumpkin with the seeds and the other ingredients, pulse well, divide into bowls and serve a party spread.

Nutrition facts per serving: calories 162, fat 12.7, fiber 2.3, carbs 9.7, protein 5.5

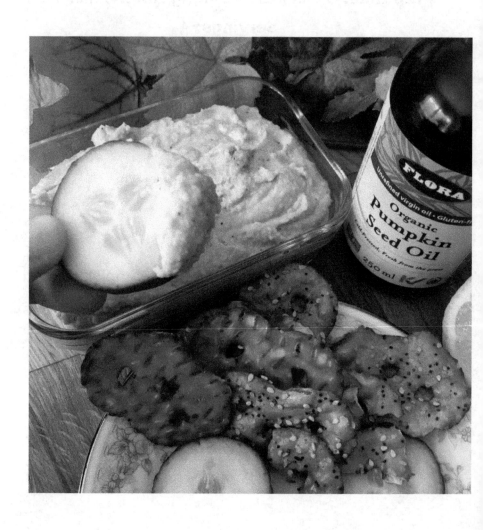

Dill Spinach Spread

Prep time: 10 minutes I **Cooking time:** 20 minutes I

Servings: 4

Ingredients:

- 1 pound spinach, chopped
- 1 cup coconut cream
- 1 cup mozzarella, shredded
- A pinch of black pepper
- 1 tablespoon dill, chopped

Directions:

1. In a baking pan, combine the spinach with the cream and the other ingredients, stir well, introduce in the oven and bake at 400 degrees F for 20 minutes.
2. Divide into bowls and serve.

Nutrition facts per serving: calories 186, fat 14.8, fiber 4.4, carbs 8.4, protein 8.8

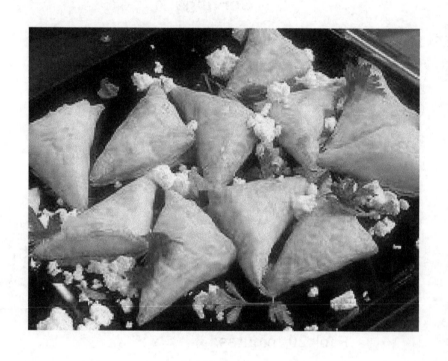

Cilantro Salsa

Prep time: 5 minutes I **Cooking time:** 0 minutes I

Servings: 4

Ingredients:

- 1 red onion, chopped
- 1 cup black olives, pitted and halved
- 1 cucumber, cubed
- ¼ cup cilantro, chopped
- A pinch of black pepper
- 2 tablespoons lime juice

Directions:

1. In a bowl, combine the olives with the cucumber and the rest of the ingredients, toss and serve cold as a snack.

Nutrition facts per serving: calories 64, fat 3.7, fiber 2.1, carbs 8.4, protein 1.1

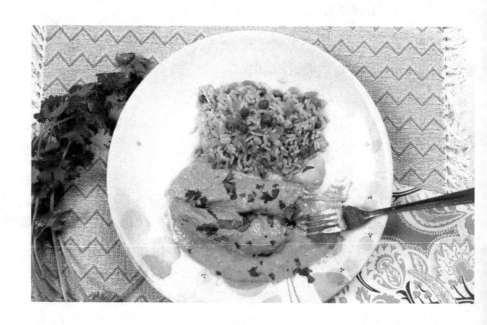

Beets Dip

Prep time: 5 minutes I **Cooking time:** 25 minutes I

Servings: 4

Ingredients:

- 2 tablespoons olive oil
- 1 red onion, chopped
- 2 tablespoons chives, chopped
- A pinch of black pepper
- 1 beet, peeled and chopped
- 8 ounces cream cheese
- 1 cup coconut cream

Directions:

1. Heat up a pan with the oil over medium heat, add the onion and sauté for 5 minutes.
2. Add the rest of the ingredients, and cook everything for 20 minutes more stirring often.
3. Transfer the mix to a blender, pulse well, divide into bowls and serve.

Nutrition facts per serving: calories 418, fat 41.2, fiber 2.5, carbs 10, protein 6.4

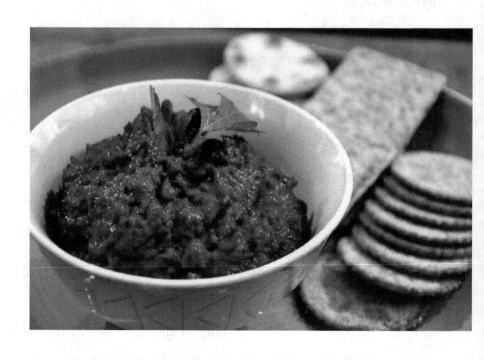

Balsamic Cucumber Bowls

Prep time: 5 minutes I **Cooking time:** 0 minutes I
Servings: 4

Ingredients:

- 1 pound cucumbers cubed
- 1 avocado, peeled, pitted and cubed
- 1 tablespoon capers, drained
- 1 tablespoon chives, chopped
- 1 small red onion, cubed
- 1 tablespoon olive oil
- 1 tablespoon balsamic vinegar

Directions:

1. In a bowl, combine the cucumbers with the avocado and the other ingredients, toss, divide into small cups and serve.

Nutrition facts per serving: calories 132, fat 4.4, fiber 4, carbs 11.6, protein 4.5

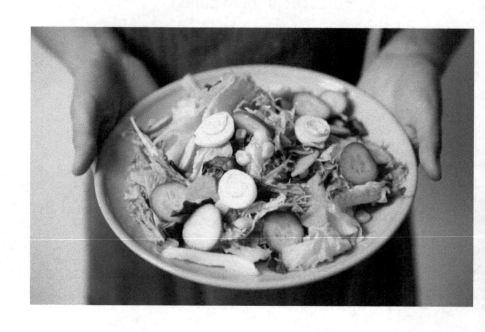

Lemon Chives Chickpeas Dip

Prep time: 5 minutes I **Cooking time:** 0 minutes I

Servings: 4

Ingredients:

- 1 tablespoon olive oil
- 1 tablespoon lemon juice
- 1 tablespoon sesame seeds paste
- 2 tablespoons chives, chopped
- 2 spring onions, chopped
- 2 cups chickpeas, cooked

Directions:

1. In your blender, combine the chickpeas with the oil and the other ingredients except the chives, pulse well, divide into bowls, sprinkle the chives on top and serve.

Nutrition facts per serving: calories 280, fat 13.3, fiber 5.5, carbs 14.8, protein 6.2

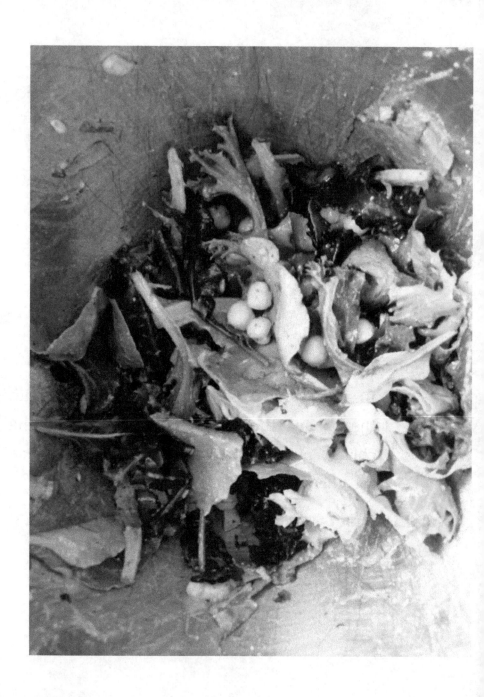

Creamy Olives Spread

Prep time: 4 minutes I **Cooking time:** 0 minutes I

Servings: 4

Ingredients:

- 2 cups black olives, pitted and chopped
- 1 cup mint, chopped
- 2 tablespoons avocado oil
- ½ cup coconut cream
- ¼ cup lime juice
- A pinch of black pepper

Directions:

1. In your blender, combine the olives with the mint and the other ingredients, pulse well, divide into bowls and serve.

Nutrition facts per serving: calories 287, fat 13.3, fiber 4.7, carbs 17.4, protein 2.4

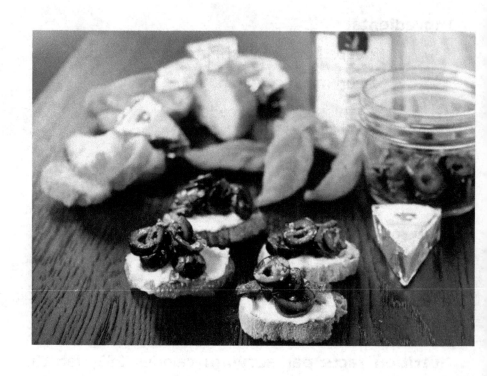

Onions Dip

Prep time: 5 minutes I **Cooking time:** 0 minutes I

Servings: 4

Ingredients:

- 4 spring onions, chopped
- 1 shallot, minced
- 1 tablespoon lime juice
- A pinch of black pepper
- 2 ounces mozzarella cheese, shredded
- 1 cup coconut cream
- 1 tablespoon parsley, chopped

Directions:

1. In a blender, combine the spring onions with the shallot and the other ingredients, pulse well, divide into bowls and serve as a party dip.

Nutrition facts per serving: calories 271, fat 15.3, fiber 5, carbs 15.9, protein 6.9

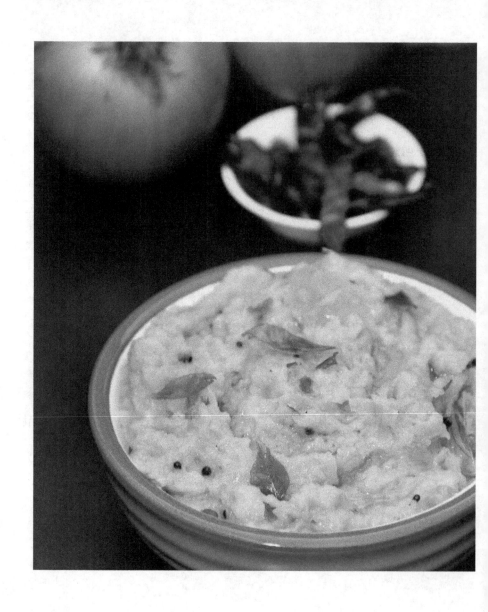

Pine Nuts Dip

Prep time: 5 minutes I **Cooking time:** 0 minutes I

Servings: 4

Ingredients:

- 8 ounces coconut cream
- 1 tablespoon pine nuts, chopped
- 2 tablespoons parsley, chopped
- A pinch of black pepper

Directions:

1. In a bowl, combine the cream with the pine nuts and the rest of the ingredients, whisk well, divide into bowls and serve.

Nutrition facts per serving: calories 281, fat 13, fiber 4.8, carbs 16, protein 3.56

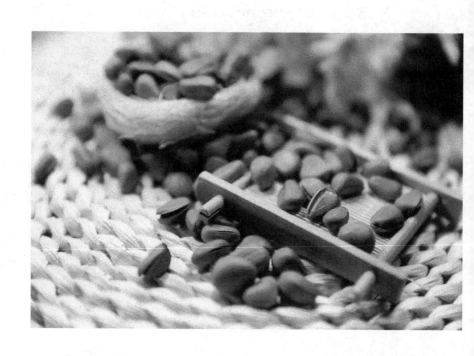

Arugula Salsa

Prep time: 5 minutes I **Cooking time:** 0 minutes I

Servings: 4

Ingredients:

- 4 scallions, chopped
- 2 tomatoes, cubed
- 4 cucumbers, cubed
- 1 tablespoon balsamic vinegar
- 1 cup baby arugula leaves
- 2 tablespoons lemon juice
- 2 tablespoons olive oil
- A pinch of black pepper

Directions:

1. In a bowl, combine the scallions with the tomatoes and the other ingredients, toss, divide into small bowls and serve as a snack.

Nutrition facts per serving: calories 139, fat 3.8, fiber 4.5, carbs 14, protein 5.4

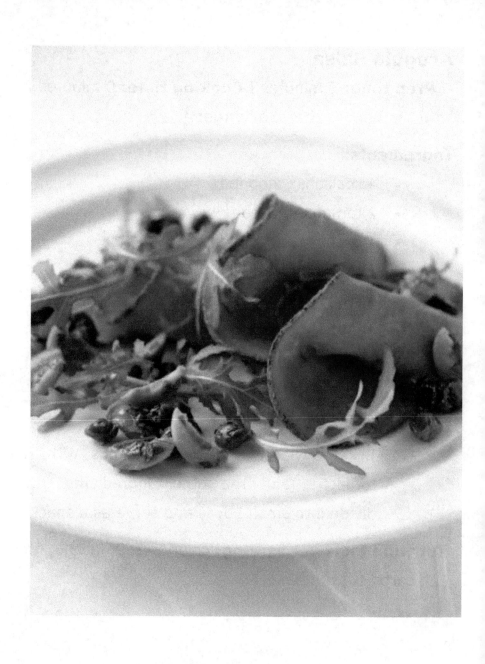

Creamy Cheese Spread

Prep time: 5 minutes

Cooking time: 0 minutes

Servings: 6

Ingredients:

- 1 tablespoon mint, chopped
- 1 tablespoon oregano, chopped
- 10 ounces cream cheese
- ½ cup ginger, sliced
- 2 tablespoons coconut aminos

Directions:

1. In your blender, combine the cream cheese with the ginger and the other ingredients, pulse well, divide into small cups and serve.

Nutrition facts per serving: calories 388, fat 15.4, fiber 6, carbs 14.3, protein 6

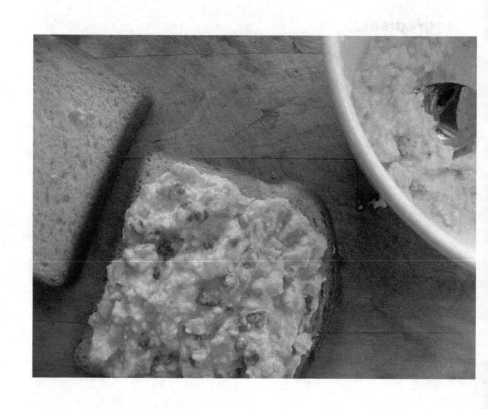

Yogurt Dip

Prep time: 5 minutes I **Cooking time:** 0 minutes I

Servings: 4

Ingredients:

- 3 cups non-fat yogurt
- 2 spring onions, chopped
- 1 teaspoon sweet paprika
- ¼ cup almonds, chopped
- ¼ cup dill, chopped

Directions:

1. In a bowl, combine the yogurt with the onions and the other ingredients, whisk, divide into bowls and serve.

Nutrition facts per serving: calories 181, fat 12.2, fiber 6, carbs 14,1, protein 7

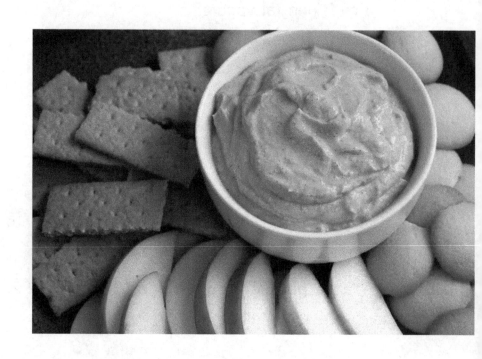

Cauliflower and Olives Salsa

Prep time: 5 minutes I **Cooking time:** 0 minutes I

Servings: 4

Ingredients:

- 1 pound cauliflower florets, blanched
- 1 cup kalamata olives, pitted and halved
- 1 cup cherry tomatoes, halved
- 1 tablespoon olive oil
- 1 tablespoon lime juice
- A pinch of black pepper

Directions:

1. In a bowl, combine the cauliflower with the olives and the other ingredients, toss and serve.

Nutrition facts per serving: calories 139, fat 4, fiber 3.6, carbs 5.5, protein 3.4

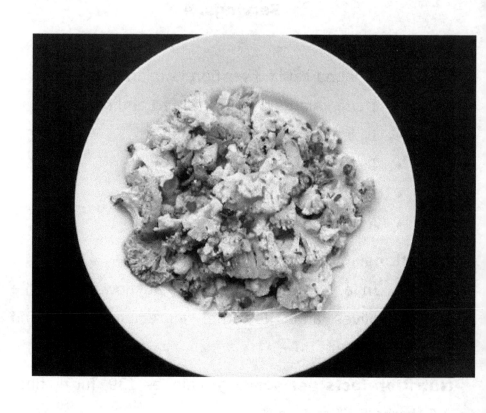

Shrimp Dip

Prep time: 5 minutes I **Cooking time:** 0 minutes I

Servings: 4

Ingredients:

- 8 ounces coconut cream
- 1 pound shrimp, cooked, peeled, deveined and chopped
- 2 tablespoons dill, chopped
- 2 spring onions, chopped
- 1 tablespoon cilantro, chopped
- A pinch of black pepper

Directions:

1. In a bowl, combine the shrimp with the cream and the other ingredients, whisk and serve as a party spread.

Nutrition facts per serving: calories 362, fat 14.3, fiber 6, carbs 14.6, protein 5.9

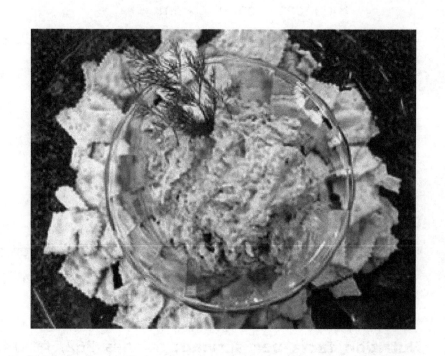

Peach Bowls

Prep time: 4 minutes I **Cooking time:** 0 minutes I

Servings: 4

Ingredients:

- 4 peaches, stones removed and cubed
- 1 cup kalamata olives, pitted and halved
- 1 avocado, pitted, peeled and cubed
- 1 cup cherry tomatoes, halved
- 1 tablespoon olive oil
- 1 tablespoon lime juice
- 1 tablespoon cilantro, chopped

Directions:

1. In a bowl, combine the peaches with the olives and the other ingredients, toss well and serve cold.

Nutrition facts per serving: calories 200, fat 7.5, fiber 5, carbs 13.3, protein 4.9

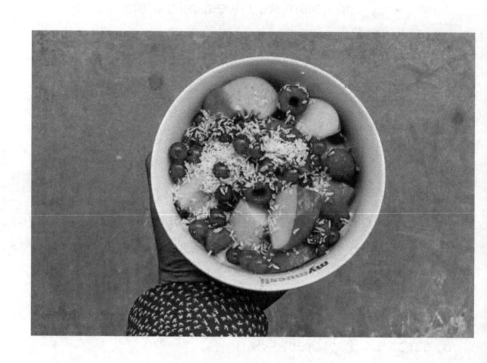

Carrot Bites

Prep time: 10 minutes I **Cooking time:** 20 minutes I

Servings: 4

Ingredients:

- 4 carrots, thinly sliced
- 2 tablespoons olive oil
- A pinch of black pepper
- 1 teaspoon sweet paprika
- ½ teaspoon turmeric powder
- A pinch of red pepper flakes

Directions:

1. In a bowl, combine the carrot chips with the oil and the other ingredients and toss.
2. Spread the chips on a lined baking sheet, bake at 400 degrees F for 25 minutes, divide into bowls and serve as a snack.

Nutrition facts per serving: calories 180, fat 3, fiber 3.3, carbs 5.8, protein 1.3

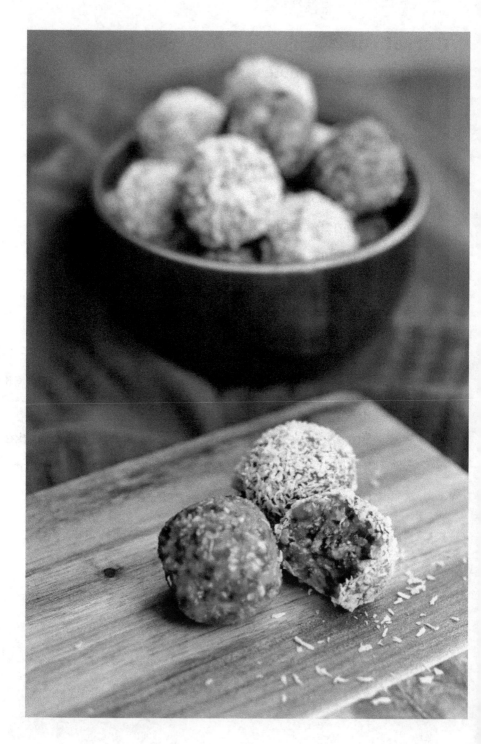

Asparagus Bites

Prep time: 4 minutes I **Cooking time:** 20 minutes I
Servings: 4

Ingredients:

- 2 tablespoons coconut oil, melted
- 1 pound asparagus, trimmed and halved
- 1 teaspoon garlic powder
- 1 teaspoon rosemary, dried
- 1 teaspoon chili powder

Directions:

1. In a bowl, mix the asparagus with the oil and the other ingredients, toss, spread on a lined baking sheet and bake at 400 degrees F for 20 minutes.
2. Divide into bowls and serve cold as a snack.

Nutrition facts per serving: calories 170, fat 4.3, fiber 4, carbs 7, protein 4.5

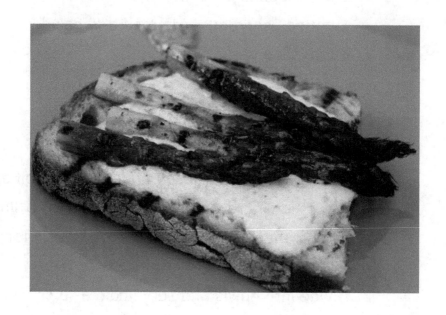

Figs Snack

Prep time: 4 minutes I **Cooking time:** 12 minutes I

Servings: 4

Ingredients:

- 8 figs, halved
- 1 tablespoon avocado oil
- 1 teaspoon nutmeg, ground

Directions:

1. In a roasting pan combine the figs with the oil and the nutmeg, toss, and bake at 400 degrees F for 12 minutes.
2. Divide the figs into small bowls and serve as a snack.

Nutrition facts per serving: calories 180, fat 4.3, fiber 2, carbs 2, protein 3.2

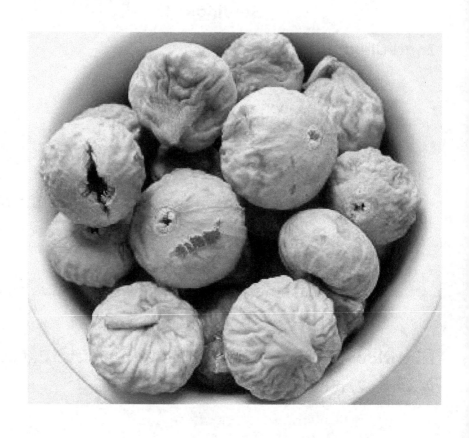

Cabbage Salsa

Prep time: 5 minutes I **Cooking time:** 6 minutes I

Servings: 4

Ingredients:

- 2 cups red cabbage, shredded
- 1 pound shrimp, peeled and deveined
- 1 tablespoon olive oil
- A pinch of black pepper
- 2 spring onions, chopped
- 1 cup tomatoes, cubed
- ½ teaspoon garlic powder

Directions:

1. Heat up a pan with the oil over medium heat, add the shrimp, toss and cook for 3 minutes on each side.
2. In a bowl, combine the cabbage with the shrimp and the other ingredients, toss, divide into small bowls and serve.

Nutrition facts per serving: calories 225, fat 9.7, fiber 5.1, carbs 11.4, protein 4.5

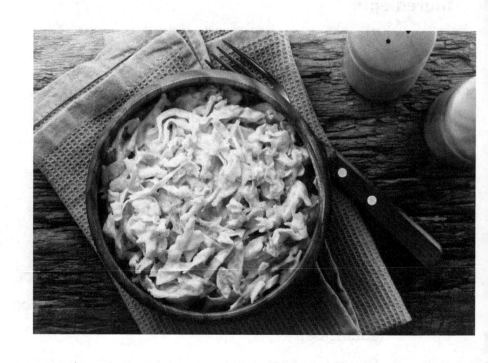

Coriander Avocado Wedges

Prep time: 5 minutes I **Cooking time:** 10 minutes I

Servings: 4

Ingredients:

- 2 avocados, peeled, pitted and cut into wedges
- 1 tablespoon avocado oil
- 1 tablespoon lime juice
- 1 teaspoon coriander, ground

Directions:

1. Spread the avocado wedges on a lined baking sheet, add the oil and the other ingredients, toss, and bake at 300 degrees F for 10 minutes.
2. Divide into cups and serve as a snack.

Nutrition facts per serving: calories 212, fat 20.1, fiber 6.9, carbs 9.8, protein 2

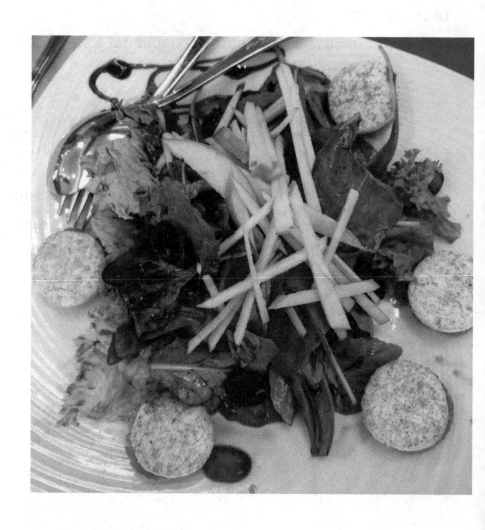

Lemon Dip

Ingredients:

- 1 cup cream cheese
- Black pepper to the taste
- ½ cup lemon juice
- 1 tablespoon cilantro, chopped
- 3 garlic cloves, chopped

Directions:

1. In your food processor, mix the cream cheese with the lemon juice and the other ingredients, pulse well, divide into bowls and serve.

Nutrition facts per serving: calories 213, fat 20.5, fiber 0.2, carbs 2.8, protein 4.8

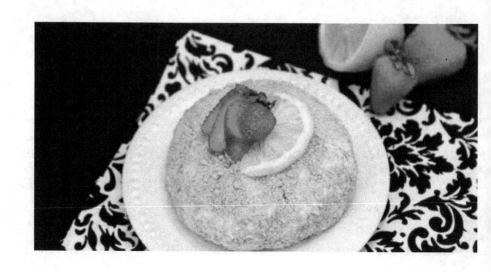

Coconut Sweet Potato Spread

Prep time: 10 minutes I **Cooking time:** 40 minutes I
Servings: 4

Ingredients:

- 1 cup sweet potatoes, peeled and cubed
- 1 tablespoon veggie stock
- Cooking spray
- 2 tablespoons coconut cream
- 2 teaspoons rosemary, dried
- Black pepper to the taste

Directions:

1. In a baking pan, combine the potatoes with the stock and the other ingredients, stir, bake at 365 degrees F for 40 minutes, transfer to your blender, pulse well, divide into small bowls and serve

Nutrition facts per serving: calories 65, fat 2.1, fiber 2, carbs 11.3, protein 0.8

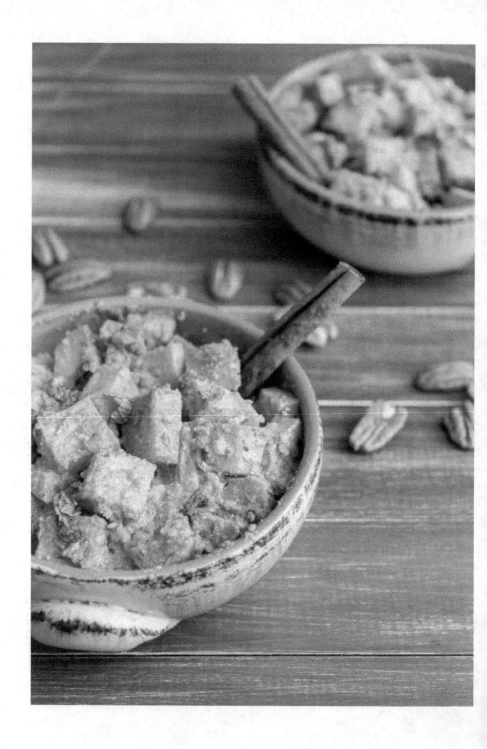

Balsamic Salsa

Prep time: 5 minutes I **Cooking time:** 0 minutes I

Servings: 4

Ingredients:

- 1 cup black beans, cooked
- 1 cup red kidney beans, cooked
- 1 teaspoon balsamic vinegar
- 1 cup cherry tomatoes, cubed
- 1 tablespoon olive oil
- 2 shallots, chopped

Directions:

1. In a bowl, combine the beans with the vinegar and the other ingredients, toss and serve as a party snack.

Nutrition facts per serving: calories 362, fat 4.8, fiber 14.9, carbs 61, protein 21.4

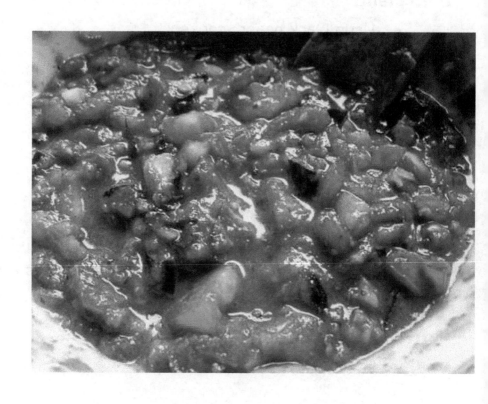

Green Olives Salsa

Prep time: 10 minutes I **Cooking time:** 10 minutes I

Servings: 4

Ingredients:

- 1 pound green beans, trimmed and halved
- 1 tablespoon olive oil
- 2 teaspoons capers, drained
- 6 ounces green olives, pitted and sliced
- 4 garlic cloves, minced
- 1 tablespoon lime juice
- 1 tablespoon oregano, chopped
- Black pepper to the taste

Directions:

1. Heat up a pan with the oil over medium-high heat, add the garlic and the green beans, toss and cook for 3 minutes.
2. Add the rest of the ingredients, toss, cook for another 7 minutes, divide into small cups and serve cold.

Nutrition facts per serving: calories 111, fat 6.7, fiber 5.6, carbs 13.2, protein 2.9

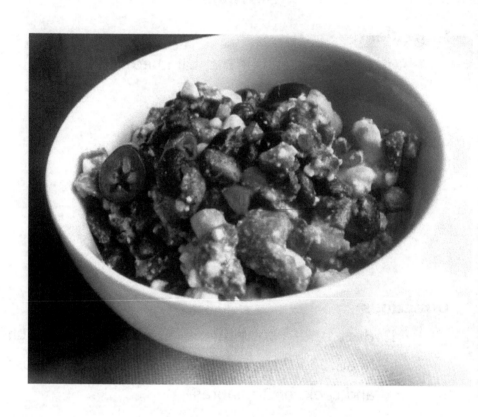

Carrot and Walnuts Spread

Prep time: 10 minutes I **Cooking time:** 30 minutes I

Servings: 4

Ingredients:

- 1 pound carrots, peeled and chopped
- ½ cup walnuts, chopped
- 2 cups veggie stock
- 1 cup coconut cream
- 1 tablespoon rosemary, chopped
- 1 teaspoon garlic powder
- ¼ teaspoon smoked paprika

Directions:

1. In a small pot, mix the carrots with the stock, walnuts and the other ingredients except the cream and the rosemary, stir, bring to a boil over medium heat, cook for 30 minutes, drain and transfer to a blender.
2. Add the cream, blend the mix well, divide into bowls, sprinkle the rosemary on top and serve.

Nutrition facts per serving: calories 201, fat 8.7, fiber 3.4, carbs 7.8, protein 7.7

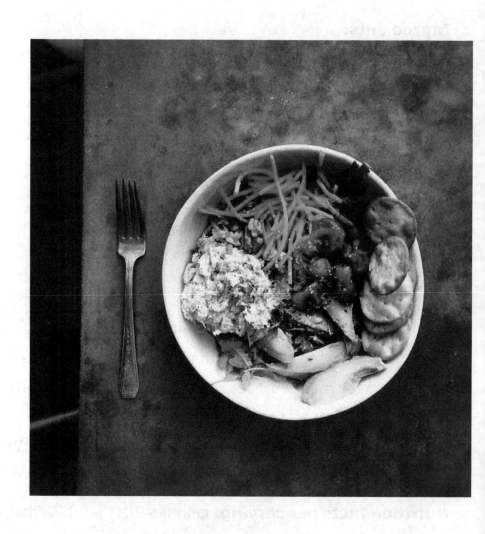

Garlic Tomato Spread

Prep time: 10 minutes I **Cooking time:** 10 minutes I

Servings: 4

Ingredients:

- 1 pound tomatoes, peeled and chopped
- ½ cup garlic, minced
- 2 tablespoons olive oil
- A pinch of black pepper
- 2 shallots, chopped
- 1 teaspoon thyme, dried

Directions:

1. Heat up a pan with the oil over medium-high heat, add the garlic and the shallots, stir and sauté for 2 minutes.
2. Add the tomatoes and the other ingredients, cook for 8 minutes more and transfer to a blender.
3. Pulse well, divide into small cups and serve as a snack.

Nutrition facts per serving: calories 232, fat 11.3, fiber 3.9, carbs 7.9, protein 4.5

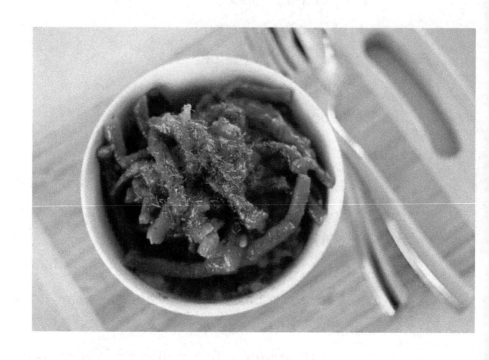

Salmon and Cucumber Wraps

Prep time: 10 minutes I **Cooking time:** 0 minutes I

Servings: 4

Ingredients:

- 6 ounces smoked salmon, skinless and thinly sliced
- 1 red bell pepper, cut into strips
- 1 cucumber, cut into strips
- 2 tablespoons coconut cream

Directions:

1. Place the smoked salmon slices on a working surface, spread the coconut cream on each, divide the cucumber and the bell pepper strips on each slide, roll and serve as a snack.

Nutrition facts per serving: calories 120, fat 6, fiber 6, carbs 12, protein 6

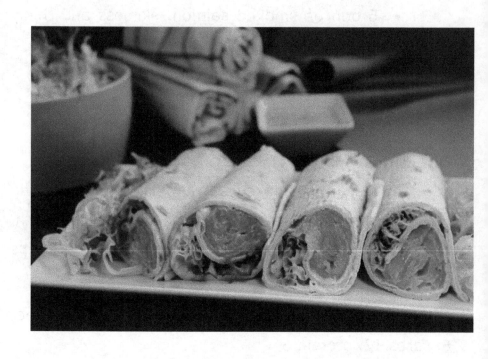

Garlic Mussels and Quinoa

Prep time: 10 minutes I **Cooking time:** 12 minutes I

Servings: 4

Ingredients:

- 1 pound mussels, scrubbed
- 2 cups quinoa, cooked
- ½ cup chicken soup
- 1 teaspoon red pepper flakes, crushed
- 1 teaspoon hot paprika
- 2 garlic cloves, minced
- 2 tablespoons parsley, chopped
- 2 tablespoons avocado oil
- 1 yellow onion, chopped
- A pinch of salt and black pepper

Directions:

1. Heat up a pan with the oil over medium heat, add the onion and the garlic and sauté for 2 minutes.
2. Add the mussels, quinoa and the other ingredients, toss, cook over medium heat for 10 minutes more, divide into small bowls and serve.

Nutrition facts per serving: calories 150, fat 3, fiber 3, carbs 6, protein 8

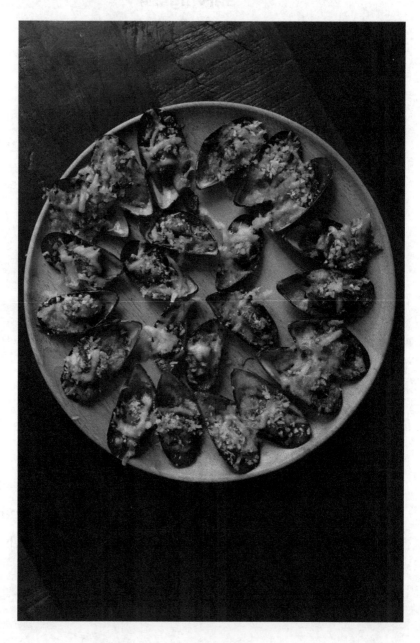

Tuna Bites

Prep time: 10 minutes I **Cooking time:** 10 minutes I
Servings: 4

Ingredients:

- 1 pound tuna fillets, boneless, skinless and cubed
- 2 tablespoons olive oil
- 4 scallions, chopped
- Juice of 1 lime
- 1 teaspoon sweet paprika
- 1 teaspoon turmeric powder
- 2 tablespoons coconut aminos
- A pinch of salt and black pepper

Directions:

1. Heat up a pan with the oil over medium heat, add the scallions and sauté for 2 minutes.
2. Add the tuna bites and cook them for 2 minutes on each side.
3. Add the remaining ingredients, toss gently, cook everything for 4 minutes more, arrange everything on a platter and serve.

Nutrition facts per serving: calories 210, fat 7, fiber 6, carbs 6, protein 7

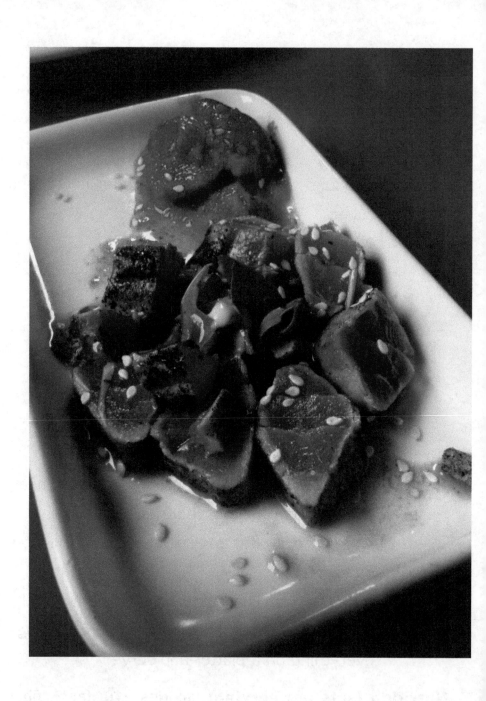

Berries Salsa

Prep time: 10 minutes I **Cooking time:** 0 minutes I

Servings: 4

Ingredients:

- 1 pound cherry tomatoes, cubed
- 1 cup blackberries
- ½ cup strawberries
- 2 tablespoons avocado oil
- 4 scallions, chopped
- 2 tablespoons garlic powder
- A pinch of salt and black pepper
- ½ tablespoon mint, chopped
- 1 tablespoon chives, chopped

Directions:

1. In a bowl, combine the tomatoes with the blackberries, strawberries and the other ingredients, toss, divide into small bowls and serve really cold.

Nutrition facts per serving: calories 60, fat 3, fiber 2, carbs 6, protein 7

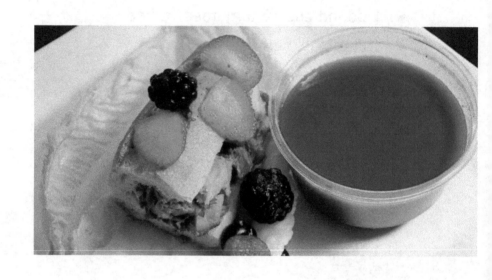

Tomato Dip

Prep time: 10 minutes I **Cooking time:** 12 minutes I

Servings: 6

Ingredients:

- 1 pound tomatoes, chopped
- 2 carrots, grated
- 4 ounces coconut cream
- A pinch of salt and black pepper
- 1 teaspoon chili powder
- Cooking spray

Directions:

1. In a pan, combine the tomatoes with the carrots and the other ingredients, toss and cook over medium heat for 12 minutes.
2. Blend using an immersion blender, divide into small bowls and serve as a party dip.

Nutrition facts per serving: calories 150, fat 4, fiber 6, carbs 14, protein 6

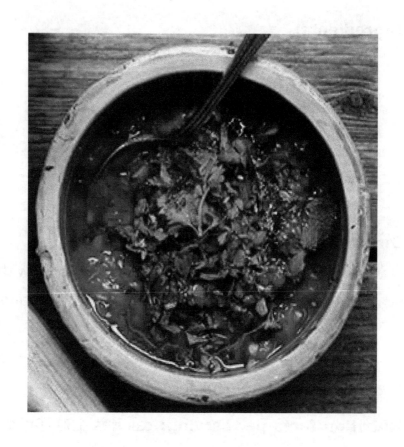

Cayenne Avocado Bites

Prep time: 10 minutes I **Cooking time:** 0 minutes I

Servings: 2

Ingredients:

- 2 avocados, halved, pitted and cubed
- ½ pound shrimp, cooked, peeled and deveined
- A pinch of salt and black pepper
- 1 tablespoon lemon juice
- 2 tablespoons olive oil
- 1 teaspoon cayenne pepper
- ½ teaspoon rosemary, dried
- ½ teaspoon oregano, dried
- 1 teaspoon sweet paprika

Directions:

1. In a bowl, combine the avocados with the shrimp, salt, pepper and the other ingredients, toss, divide into small bowls and serve.

Nutrition facts per serving: calories 160, fat 10, fiber 7, carbs 12, protein 7

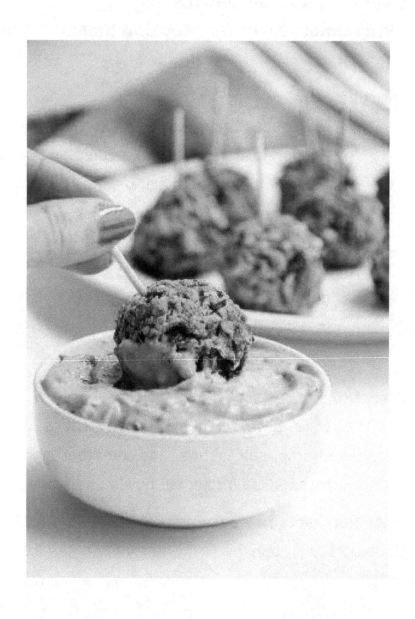

Basil Radish Snack

Prep time: 5 minutes I **Cooking time:** 25 minutes I
Servings: 4

Ingredients:

- 1 pound radishes, cut into wedges
- 2 tablespoons olive oil
- ½ teaspoon garam masala
- ½ teaspoon oregano, dried
- ½ teaspoon basil, dried
- Salt and black pepper to the taste
- 1 tablespoon chives, chopped

Directions:

1. Spread the radishes on a baking sheet lined with parchment paper, add the oil, garam masala and the other ingredients, toss and bake at 420 degrees F for 25 minutes.
2. Divide the radish bites into bowls and serve as a snack.

Nutrition facts per serving: calories 30, fat 1, fiber 2, carbs 7, protein 1

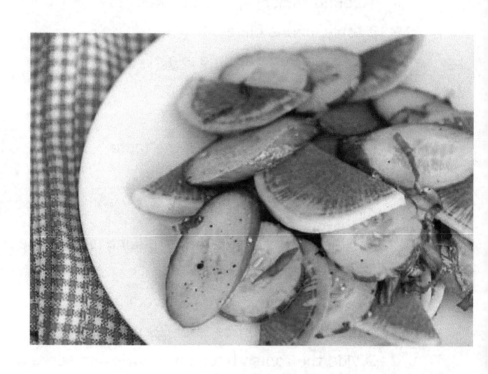

Radish Dip

Prep time: 5 minutes I **Cooking time:** 0 minutes I

Servings: 4

Ingredients:

- 2 avocados, pitted, peeled and chopped
- 1 cup radishes, chopped
- 1 cup coconut cream
- 4 spring onions, chopped
- 1 tablespoon lemon juice
- A pinch of salt and black pepper
- 1 tablespoon avocado oil

Directions:

1. In a blender, combine the avocados with the radishes and the other ingredients, pulse well, divide into bowls and serve as a party dip.

Nutrition facts per serving: calories 162, fat 8, fiber 4, carbs 6, protein 6

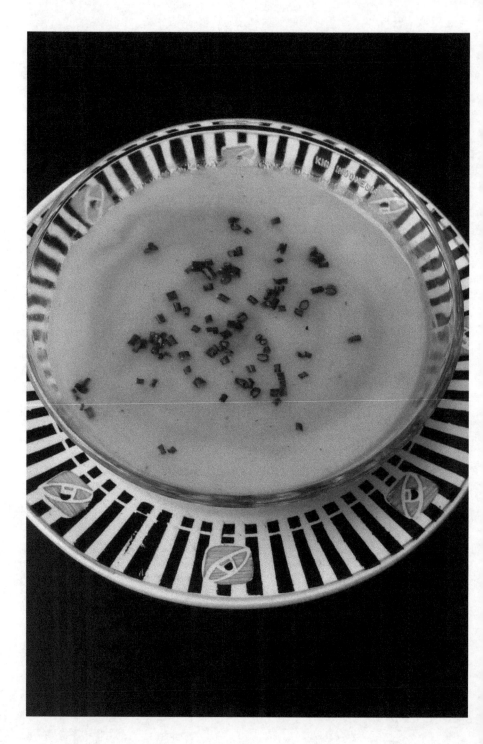

Ginger Olives Salsa

Prep time: 10 minutes I **Cooking time:** 0 minutes I

Servings: 6

Ingredients:

- 1 teaspoon cumin seeds
- 1 tablespoon avocado oil
- 2 oranges, peeled and cut into segments
- 1 cup kalamata olives, pitted and halved
- 1 tablespoon oregano, chopped
- 1 tablespoon chives, chopped
- 1 tablespoon balsamic vinegar
- ½ tablespoon ginger, grated
- ½ teaspoon fennel seeds

Directions:

1. In a bowl, combine the oranges with the olives, cumin and the other ingredients, toss, keep in the fridge for 10 minutes, divide into small bowls and serve.

Nutrition facts per serving: calories 120, fat 1, fiber 3, carbs 5, protein 9

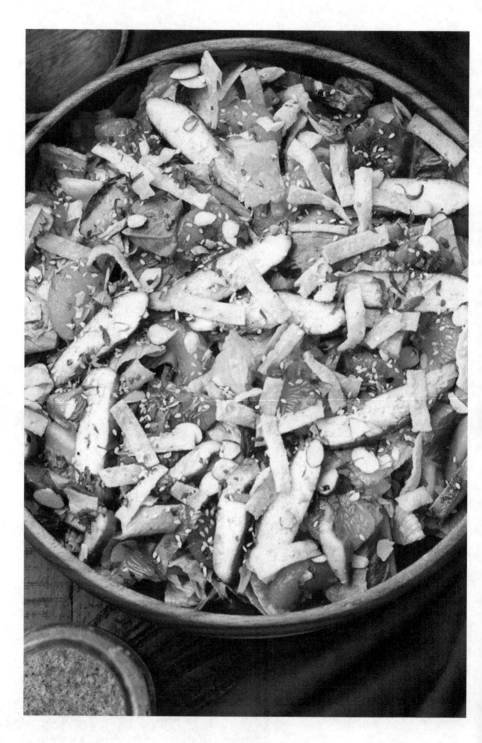

Basil Peppers Salsa

Prep time: 5 minutes I **Cooking time:** 0 minutes I
Servings: 4

Ingredients:

- 1 tablespoon olive oil
- 2 red bell peppers, cut into thin strips
- 2 green bell peppers, cut into strips
- 1 cup radishes, cubed
- 2 tablespoons balsamic vinegar
- 1 tablespoon ginger, grated
- 1 teaspoon chili powder
- 1 tablespoon lemon juice
- A pinch of salt and black pepper
- 1 tablespoon basil, chopped

Directions:

1. In a bowl, combine the bell peppers with the radishes, the oil and the other ingredients, toss, divide into small bowls and serve as a party salsa.

Nutrition facts per serving: calories 107, fat 4, fiber 2, carbs 6, protein 6

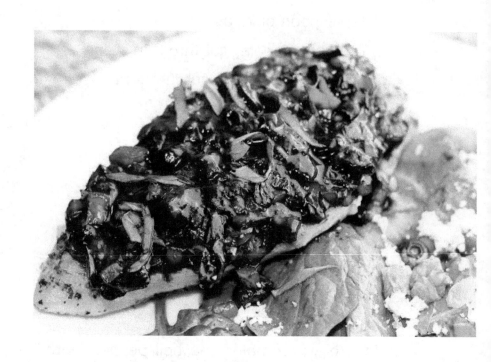

Beans Dip

Prep time: 10 minutes I **Cooking time:** 20 minutes I

Servings: 6

Ingredients:

- 2 cups red kidney beans, cooked
- 2 tablespoons olive oil
- 1 yellow onion, chopped
- ½ cup chicken stock
- ½ cup coconut cream
- ¼ teaspoon oregano, dried
- ¼ teaspoon garlic powder
- ¼ teaspoon onion powder
- Salt and black pepper to the taste
- 1 tablespoon chives, chopped

Directions:

1. Heat up a pan with the oil over medium heat, add the onion and sauté for 5 minutes.
2. Add the stock, oregano and the other ingredients except the cream and the chives, stir, and cook over medium heat for 15 minutes more.
3. Add the cream, blend the mix using an immersion blender, divide into bowls and serve with the chives sprinkled on top.

Nutrition facts per serving: calories 302, fat 10.2, fiber 10.2, carbs 40.7, protein 14.6

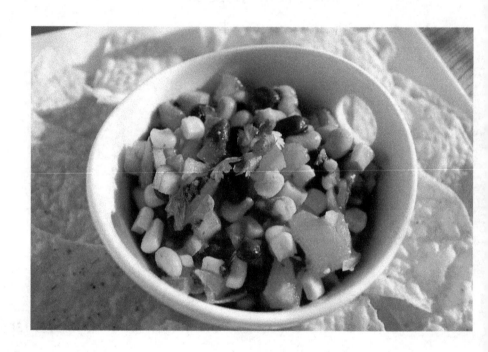

Mint Dip

Prep time: 10 minutes I **Cooking time:** 0 minutes I

Servings: 4

Ingredients:

- 2 avocados, pitted, peeled and chopped
- 1 cup cherry tomatoes, chopped
- 1 tablespoon lemon juice
- 2 tablespoons coconut oil
- 1 teaspoon chili powder
- ½ cup mint, chopped
- A pinch of salt and black pepper

Directions:

1. In a blender, mix the tomatoes with the avocado and the other ingredients, pulse well, divide into small bowls and serve as a party dip.

Nutrition facts per serving: calories 150, fat 7, fiber 6, carbs 8.8, protein 6

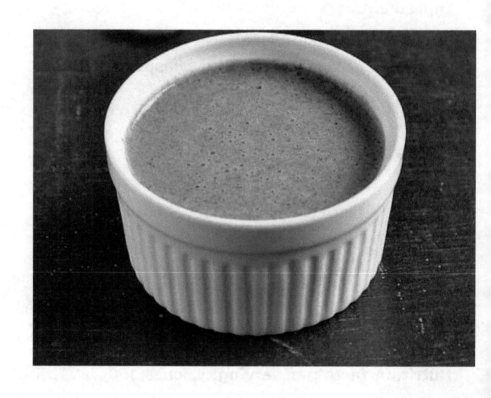

Shrimp and Watermelon Bowls

Prep time: 10 minutes I **Cooking time:** 0 minutes I

Servings: 4

Ingredients:

- 2 tablespoons avocado oil
- 4 scallions, chopped
- 1 pound shrimp, cooked, deveined and peeled
- 1 cup watermelon, peeled and cubed
- ½ cup strawberries
- 2 tablespoons lemon juice
- A pinch of cayenne pepper
- 1 tablespoon balsamic vinegar

Directions:

1. In a bowl, combine the shrimp with the watermelon, scallions and the other ingredients, toss, divide into smaller bowls and serve.

Nutrition facts per serving: calories 205, fat 12, fiber 2, carbs 9, protein 8

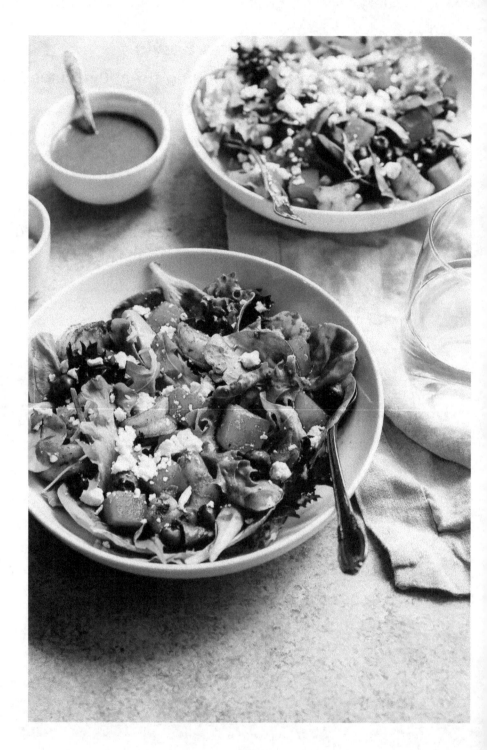

Cayenne Dip

Prep time: 10 minutes I **Cooking time:** 0 minutes I

Servings: 4

Ingredients:

- 1 avocado, pitted, peeled and chopped
- 1 red chili pepper, minced
- 1 cup blackberries
- ½ cup blueberries
- A pinch of cayenne pepper
- 2 tablespoons lemon juice

Directions:

1. In a blender, combine the avocado with the berries and the other ingredients, pulse well, divide into small bowls and serve as a party dip.

Nutrition facts per serving: calories 120, fat 2, fiber 2, carbs 7, protein 4

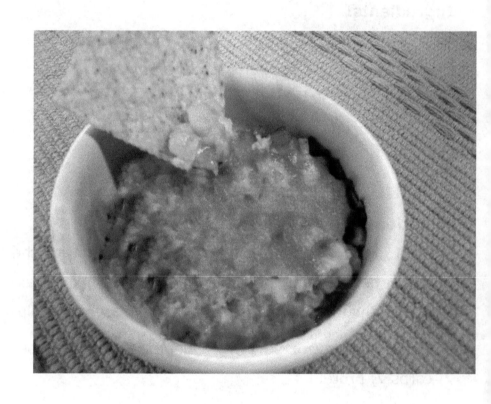

Lemon Triangles

Prep time: 5 minutes I **Cooking time:** 25 minutes I

Servings: 4

Ingredients:

- 1 cup coconut flour
- A pinch of salt and black pepper
- 1 cup cilantro, chopped
- 1 teaspoon lemon zest, grated
- 1 tablespoon lemon juice
- 2 eggs, whisked
- ½ teaspoon baking powder

Directions:

1. In a bowl, mix the flour with the eggs and the other ingredients, and stir well.
2. Spread the mix on a baking sheet lined with parchment paper, cut into triangles and cook at 380 degrees F for 25 minutes.
3. Cool the squares down and serve them as a snack.

Nutrition facts per serving: calories 49, fat 2.7, fiber 1.4, carbs 2.8, protein 3.4

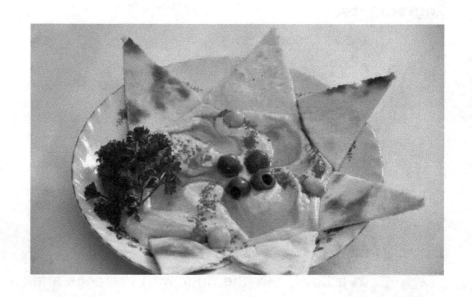

Coconut Peppers Spread

Prep time: 4 minutes I **Cooking time:** 0 minutes I

Servings: 4

Ingredients:

- 1 teaspoon turmeric powder
- 1 cup coconut cream
- 14 ounces red peppers, chopped
- Juice of ½ lemon
- 1 tablespoon chives, chopped

Directions:

1. In your blender, combine the peppers with the turmeric and the other ingredients except the chives, pulse well, divide into bowls and serve as a snack with the chives sprinkled on top.

Nutrition facts per serving: calories 183, fat 14.9, fiber 3. carbs 12.7, protein 3.4

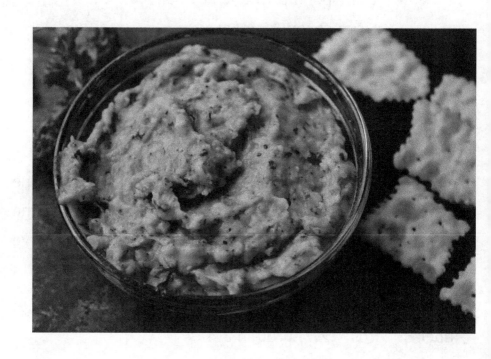

Lentils Cilantro Dip

Prep time: 5 minutes I **Cooking time:** 0 minutes I

Servings: 4

Ingredients:

- 14 ounces lentils, cooked
- Juice of 1 lemon
- 2 garlic cloves, minced
- 2 tablespoons olive oil
- ½ cup cilantro, chopped

Directions:

1. In a blender, combine the lentils with the oil and the other ingredients, pulse well, divide into bowls and serve as a party spread.

Nutrition facts per serving: calories 416, fat 8.2, fiber 30.4, carbs 60.4, protein 25.8

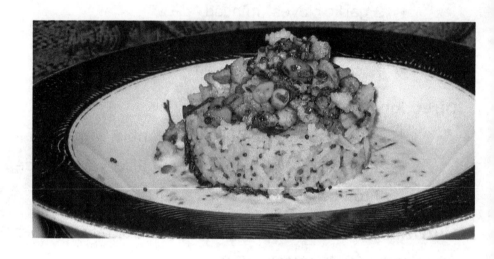

Spiced Walnuts Mix

Prep time: 5 minutes I **Cooking time:** 15 minutes I

Servings: 8

Ingredients:

- ½ teaspoon smoked paprika
- ½ teaspoon chili powder
- ½ teaspoon garlic powder
- 1 tablespoon avocado oil
- A pinch of cayenne pepper
- 14 ounces walnuts

Directions:

1. Spread the walnuts on a lined baking sheet, add the paprika and the other ingredients, toss and bake at 410 degrees F for 15 minutes.
2. Divide into bowls and serve as a snack.

Nutrition facts per serving: calories 311, fat 29.6, fiber 3.6, carbs 5.3, protein 12

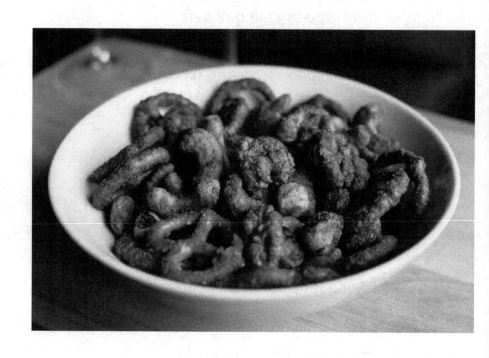

Cranberry Bites

Prep time: 3 hours and 5 minutes I **Cooking time:** 0 minutes I **Servings:** 4

Ingredients:

- 2 ounces coconut cream
- 2 tablespoons rolled oats
- 2 tablespoons coconut, shredded
- 1 cup cranberries

Directions:

1. In a blender, combine the oats with the cranberries and the other ingredients, pulse well and spread into a square pan.
2. Cut into squares and keep them in the fridge for 3 hours before serving.

Nutrition facts per serving: calories 66, fat 4.4, fiber 1.8, carbs 5.4, protein 0.8

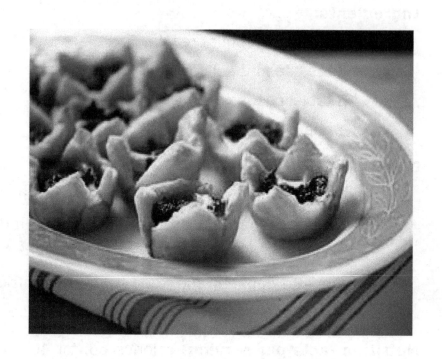

Cheddar Cauliflower Bars

Prep time: 10 minutes I **Cooking time:** 30 minutes I

Servings: 8

Ingredients:

- 2 cups whole wheat flour
- 2 teaspoons baking powder
- A pinch of black pepper
- 2 eggs, whisked
- 1 cup almond milk
- 1 cup cauliflower florets, chopped
- ½ cup cheddar, shredded

Directions:

1. In a bowl, combine the flour with the cauliflower and the other ingredients and stir well.
2. Spread into a baking tray, introduce in the oven, bake at 400 degrees F for 30 minutes, cut into bars and serve as a snack.

Nutrition facts per serving: calories 430, fat 18.1, fiber 3.7, carbs 54, protein 14.5

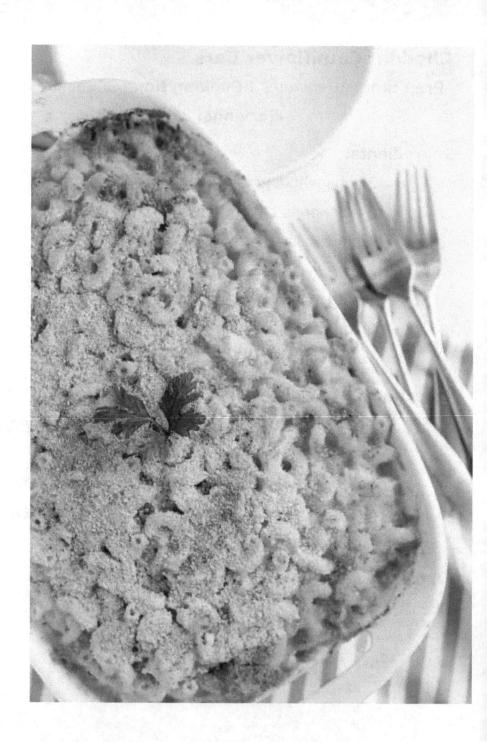

Almonds Bowls

Prep time: 5 minutes I **Cooking time:** 10 minutes I

Servings: 4

Ingredients:

- 2 cups almonds
- ¼ cup coconut, shredded
- 1 mango, peeled and cubed
- 1 cup sunflower seeds
- Cooking spray

Directions:

1. Spread the almonds, coconut, mango and sunflower seeds on a baking tray, grease with the cooking spray, toss and bake at 400 degrees F for 10 minutes.
2. Divide into bowls and serve as a snack.

Nutrition facts per serving: calories 411, fat 31.8, fiber 8.7, carbs 25.8, protein 13.3

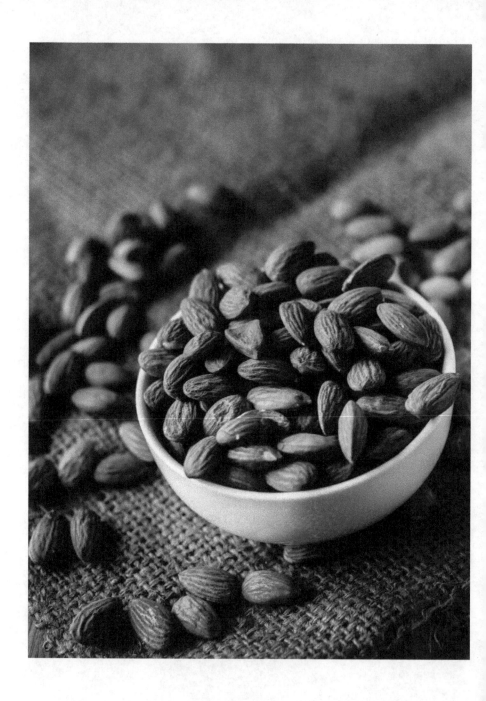

Paprika Potato Chips

Prep time: 10 minutes I **Cooking time:** 20 minutes I

Servings: 4

Ingredients:

- 4 gold potatoes, peeled and thinly sliced
- 2 tablespoons olive oil
- 1 tablespoon chili powder
- 1 teaspoon sweet paprika
- 1 tablespoon chives, chopped

Directions:

1. Spread the chips on a lined baking sheet, add the oil and the other ingredients, toss, introduce in the oven and bake at 390 degrees F for 20 minutes.
2. Divide into bowls and serve.

Nutrition facts per serving: calories 118, fat 7.4, fiber 2.9, carbs 13.4, protein 1.3

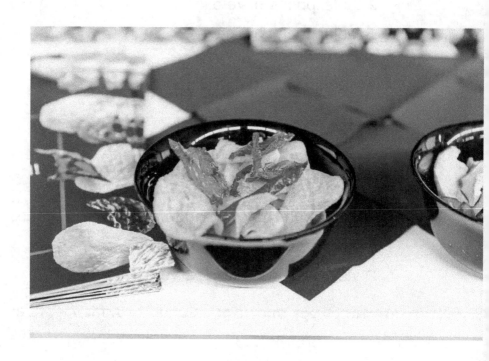

CPSIA information can be obtained
at www.ICGtesting.com
Printed in the USA
BVHW091047090621
609091BV00008B/784